7-fold Therapy

Therapy

Holistic Spiritual Medicine

Second edition 2016

New possibilities in Healing through space and time, a spiritual journey.

Healing through the middle point, based on Anthroposophy.

An addition to and an extension of my book "Holistic (veterinary) Medicine".

By
Are Simeon Thoresen DVM

MW00961640

1

7-fold way to Therapy

Holistic Spiritual Medicine

Second edition

**A Holistic View of Spiritual Medicine
based on Anthroposophy**

By

Are Simeon Thoresen, DVM

© 2016 Are Simeon Thoresen, DVM

For questions on the rights of this book please contact:

Are Thoresen
Leikvollgata 31
N-3213 Sandefjord
Email: arethore@online.no

All rights reserved. The contents of this book, both photographic and textual, may not be reproduced in any form; by print, photo print, photo transparency, microfilm, microfiche, slide or any other means, nor may it be included in any computer retrieval system without written permission from the publisher.

Remark: The author takes no responsibility for the practical use of the methods described in this book.

This book aims to give readers, professional and lay, an understanding of the *spiritual* foundations of alternative medicine, philosophy, principles and practice.

Printed version;   **ISBN :1517477662**

Electronic version;   **ISBN**

Published by Amazon

Dedicated to All
Who Seek to Heal and understand

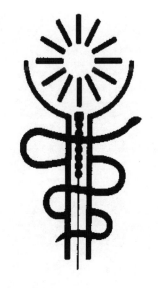

Introduction I;

My first book was written over 31 years.
During the 4 years from February 2011, until the summer of 2015, I went through a fast and deep development with many realizations, both spiritually, energetically, religiously and professionally.

The main realizations were the following;

- The hands are highly spiritual organs. They can, when the fingertips meet the blood, as in pulse diagnosis, be transformed to highways into the spiritual world, and serve as organs of initiation.
- The pulse-diagnosis is not a technique, it is a state of consciousness.
- The changes in the pulse are not happening in the physical world, but in the spiritual.
- To be able to detect pulse changes we have to be in the spiritual world.
- To enter the spiritual world we have to separate either our thinking/feeling/willing or the elements of the physical world as height/width/depth/time.
- Working with pulse-diagnosis is a way of initiation into the spiritual world.
- Most diseases (80%) in children and animals are projections from the "grown-ups", the parents.
- The projections are real pathological entities, real pathological information, real "demons".
- All symptoms (diseases) are "pathological" information, and such information is not lost easily (information is never lost).
- When we treat the excess after ordinary methods (the theory of the 5-star elemental Chinese theory) we just translocate the disease, the "excessive pathological information", which is mostly of Yang (astral) nature.
- When we treat the deficiency after the control theory of the 5-star elemental Chinese theory (as lectured by me before) we

often just translocate the disease, the "deficient pathological information", which is mostly of Yin (etheric) nature.

- If we treat the middle, the equilibrium, the mid-point between excess-Yang-astral and deficiency-Yin-etheric, we will not translocate the disease, but dissolve it.
- The so-called pathological structure is a living entity, which in old times was called a demon.

  o The Yin structures were called Ahrimanic demons.
  o The Yang structures were called Luziferic demons.

- The 5-element star system of Chinese medicine is just a construct relating to the treatment of excess and deficiency, and do not function well in finding and treating the midpoint, and therefore must be revised.
- The 6-star system is a better system to use to treat and find the midpoint.
- The mid-point is related to the Christ-consciousness, and may be found by ways of;

  o Pulse; the Christ energy, where it is felt.
  o Pulse, the controller of the deficiency relating to the 5-star (father of the father of the symptoms).
  o Pulse; the midpoint of the triangle, the trinity.
  o Anatomically; the bodily midpoint between excess (Luzifer) and deficiency (Ahriman).
  o Cranio-sacrally; the midpoint at the head between excess (Luzifer) and deficiency (Ahriman).

Thus, in the summer of 2015 I understood that my book on alternative medicine needed to be revised and updated. All the above understandings had dawned on my mind and spirit, and I felt that I had so much new information to tell the world.
I realized how much work it would take to update my >800 pages book, and did not look forward to that immense work.

The inspiration to write a new book came to me at 5 o'clock in the morning on the 3rd of September 2015, in Germany, after having twice travelled to the old mystery places of Thinking, Feeling and Willing situated in Ireland[1] in the last years before the destruction of Atlantis, and meeting the three women C, H and A, who made me aware of the cosmic Thinking, Feeling and Willing.

I suddenly understood that it was better to write a new book on **spiritual** medicine, rather than update the old one on **holistic** medicine.

I am happy here to be able to present the result of that inspiration.

Are Simeon Thoresen
Sandefjord, Norway
15th of October 2015

The disciple

all what the earth brings forth,
of bread and wine,
is now his body.
When somebody eats this,
And understand what he does,
Then he will resurrect in him.

Jens Björneboe

---

[1] *The story about that travel is told in my book "The forgotten mysteries of Atlantis", published on Amazon.com.*

Introduction II;

Treating the Middle or the Christ-point, and its effects.
(Written January 2016)

In the first edition of this book I cited a poem written by Jens Bjørneboe, called „*The disciple*". One verse of it is as follows;

The disciple

... all what the earth brings forth,
of bread and wine,
is now his body.
When somebody eats this,
And understand what he does,
Then he will resurrect in him.

Jens Björneboe

What is here said, is that the effect of the bread and wine is totally different if you ***understand*** what the eurachrist really is. Knowledge and insight change the reality, as is predicted also in quantum physics.

To understand the existence of demons and the transforming effect of the Christ-point, change the reality of the acupuncture treatment.

To be able to understand this book I have to write this second introduction.

This introduction will in some way warn the reader of this little book about the possible change his therapy will, must or may go through.

To understand what I now am going to tell you, we need to start with an experience I had many years ago, in 1983.

In the beginning of my practice I had observed that my consciousness about the life and existence of trees, of the life of nature in general, had a distinct effect on the results of my treatments.[2]

Also, I had been treating Herpes Zoster for some years, but had absolutely no results or effect on this disease. Then I read a lecture of Rudolf Steiner about the spiritual causes of Herpes Zoster, and immediately my clinical results changed from 0% to 90%, doing exactly the same treatment as before reading this lecture. I was amazed!

It seems then, that the knowledge and understanding of diseases and how to treat them is of great importance to the outcome of the treatment.

Now again this spiritual reality has stretched its hands out into my life.

Many years ago when I realized that diseases may be translocated after a "normal" treatment, in fact most of them *are* translocated, I had no idea how to avoid that. Later I learned and realized that in treating the middle or Christ-point this effect might be avoided. However, in some diseases of great importance for the patient, I was not ready to change my good-working protocol, as I feared that the effect might be lessened. So, in the diseases where I continued to use the "old" 5-element based Co-cycle treatment, the effect of the "old" treatment (after 5-elements) started to fade.
This I experienced especially when treating cancer patients. And not only I experienced this.
Also some of my students, especially those closely attached to me, experienced a significant decrease of the effect and results in treating cancer and cancer-patients.
When treating according to the 6 processes (elements), the middle- or Christ-point, the effect returned.

---

[2] *This is described in my book "Poppel" (Norwegian edition), which is translated to both English (Poplar) and German (Pappel). All three books are published on Amazon.com.*

Also within homeopathy I observed a similar effect. The good results that I previously had in cancer patients reappeared only when I used the remedies related to the fighting of the demonic entities causing cancer. Also the *"Herrings law"*[3] that is known within homeopathy will cease to be of importance if you treat after the middle point.

"Herrings law" is presented as a law of healing, which it is not. It is the law of translocation, which describes the translocation within the body, but leaves out the translocation to other entities like family, friends or animals.

This law can only be understood with the background of "Demonology".

The homeopathic remedies listed on the next page are some of those that obey to the knowledge of the middle point, the Christ-point and demonology.

3

Herrings Law. This law states that cure occurs from; a). From above downwards. b). From within outwards. c). Appearance of symptoms in reverse chronological order. This means: a); "From above downwards." Cure progresses from the head towards the lower trunk, that is to say, head symptoms clear first with regard extremities, cure spread from shoulder to fingers, or hip to toes. b); Cure starts from within outwards. Cure progresses from more important organs (e.g. liver, endocrine) to less important organs (e.g. joints). That is to say, the function of vital organ is restored before those less important to life. The end results of this externalization of disease is often the production of treatment coetaneous rash. c); "Appearance of symptoms in reverse chronological order". More recent symptoms and pathology will clear before old symptoms and pathology. The disease "back tracks" so to speak. After the more recent problems have been cleared, it is not at all uncommon for the patient to experience the transient recurrence of old symptoms and pathology which then disappears within a few weeks. Herrings Law, which is also termed the Law of Cure, is the logical inverse of the way in which chronic disease progresses both with regard to the patient himself and the ancestral history of the disease. The most important aspects of the Herrings Law are, "From within outwards" and "in reverse chronological order".

Actinides;

Actinides
Actinium
Thorium
Protactinium
Uranium
Neptunium
Plutonium
Americium
Curium
Berkelium
Californium
Einsteinium
Fermium
Mendelevium
Nobalium
Lawrencium

Lanthanides;

Lanthanium
Cerium
Praseodymium
Neodymium
Promethium
Samarium
Europium
Gadolinium
Terbium
Dysprosium
Holmium
Erbium
Thulium
Ytterbium
Lutetium

A further explanation of how to use these remedies will follow at the end of this book.

"Most diseases in children and animals are projections from the "grown-ups", the parents."

Woman, lion and horse

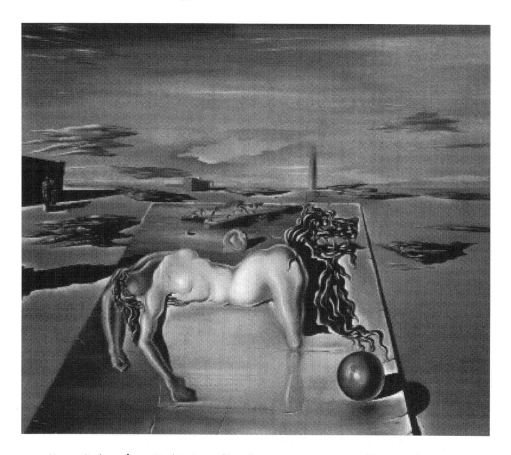

How Salvador Dali saw the humans mirror themselves in animals

Be aware of how Dali saw the etheric animals located in one direction (horse), astral animals located in the other direction (lion), and man (woman) in the middle. Here we have both the Luziferic, the Ahrimanic and the Man in the middle, as well as we see the man mirrored in the animal world. A truly ingenious picture.

Chapter one;

New insights and achievements in Pulse Diagnosis. A further deepening.
The 12 layers of the body. The importance of the heart.

For many years I lectured that the pulse was like a doorway into the energetic world, into the spiritual world.
Now I know that this is just a small part of the truth. The pulse is only the tool, by which we become aware of the observations we make in the spiritual world. The real doorway is our own mind. And that is why the preparations we make before taking the pulse are of crucial importance.

The preparations before we take the pulse are of the greatest importance.

Without these preparations we will feel nothing in the pulse. The pulse is just the tool. The mind, the soul and the spirit are the doorway.

In my first book I described the preparations as follows;

"Pulse-diagnosis is a very old method of diagnosing, used in China for thousands of years. This method may seem incredible, nonsensical or fraudulent for the western scientific mind (I must admit that based on a materialistic world-view the pulse diagnosis IS nonsensical. The diagnosis takes place in the energetic/spiritual world, not the physical). It is none of these; in skilled hands, it is a powerful diagnostic method.

Proper pulse taking requires a proper state of mind. This mind-set is similar to a form of meditation, or a state of daydreaming. Typically, a practitioner in this state is producing mainly alpha brain waves. There are at least three conditions that help a practitioner to achieve this meditative state, a state in which detachment or disassociation is crucial:

- **Not caring:** The practitioner must not have preconceptions of the causes of the disease; s/he must shed all interest, anxiety or desire to reach a diagnosis, to get paid at the end of the treatment or any other mundane matters. Many find this to be the most difficult aspect of the requirements, but this state of mind is fundamental to achieving a meditative state. Simply put, it is living in the exact moment of the pulse and of being conscious of little else.
- **Not mind wandering:** At the moment of the pulse taking, one should concentrate totally and exclusively on the patient. One's mental focus should exclude everything and everyone else that may try to enter one's mind or field of consciousness, such as being aware of the tempting sexuality of a most desirable animal handler, etc.
- **Not acting:** This is the state that some refer to as the state of fuzzy sight. It is similar to the moments when exhaustion begins to set in and the eyes gaze into the far distance. In this state, one finds it difficult to concentrate on other things. Therefore one does not act, or attains the state of not acting."

Today I will put this differently.

The main and crucial technique or tool to enter the spiritual world is to separate "something" in your soul or mind.

What is this "something"?

We are held, or imprisoned in the physical world because our soul qualities; Thinking, Feeling and Willing are linked together. This reflects also in that the different dimensions of the physical world are linked together; as height, width, depth and time (we experience these dimensions of an object at the same time).
To enter the spiritual world we have to separate either our thinking/feeling/willing or the elements of the physical world as height/width/depth/time.

The technique I will describe is used by all cultures.
As feeling is related to the depth, the easiest and best thing is to start by separating the depth from the width or height. This is done by sort of day dreaming; when you merge, or wander away in the wide expanses of the world. Many experience this state of mind during boring lectures or conversations, when you suddenly fade away and do not really hear what is said. We must, before we take the pulse, sort of fade away. Then thinking and willing are left behind, and we just feel. We do not think as "clever" as before, and we are unable to "will" anything. We feel a slight tinnitus, and the colors of the landscape change a little; a slight turning towards violet.

In the elf-school of Reykjavik, Iceland, the teachers use this technique when they prepare to speak to the elves. They fade away into the landscape, excarnate slightly, the landscape turns a little purple and then the elves appear.

Then we **are** in the spiritual world. We have then to be aware that the laws in the physical world and the spiritual world are different. In the physical world we are bound to the elements that are linked together. In the spiritual world this is not so. Time and the three dimensions are not linked. We are present exactly where our mind is. When we then concentrate on a patient, we **are** within that patient, no matter how far away the patient is.
When we go back in time, as described in chapter seven, we **are** in the past.

When this preparation is done, we concentrate on our heart. We imagine a tunnel between our own heart and the heart of the patient. Then we are connected to the spirit or energies of the patient. Then we **are** in the heart of the patient.

Between the skin and the center of the heart there are 12 layers, through which we have to penetrate. Most of my students stop at the 5th-6th-7th-8th layer, and do not enter the heart. We need a little power to enter the heart, a little bravery, a little push.

I will here refer to the 12 layers of the body;

- The outer layers (1-2) relate to the astral body
- The next (3rd-4th) to the material body (3rd being our own physical, material body, 4th parasitic material bodies)
- The 5th-6th-7th-8th relate to the etheric (the 4 ethers) body (the 7th touching the pericardium and the 8th touching the endocardium), where we leave the material world ......
- The inner layers (9th-10th-11th-12th) are within the heart, and relate to the "I"; the lower I (9th), the middle I (10th), the higher I (11th) and the cosmic I (the Christ consciousness) (12th), where we are in the middle of the heart, the lamb (ram), the Christ consciousness.

The 12 layers of the pulse

Between the skin (actually outside the skin) there are 12 layers, or depths, of which disease may be diagnosed (or treated)

12

- The outer layer (1-2) relate to the astral body
- The next (3-4) to the material body (3 being our own material body, 4. parasitic material bodies)
- The 5-6-7-8 to the etheric (the 4 ethers) body (the 7. touching the pericardium and the 8. touching the endocardium), where we leave the material world ......
- The inner (9-10-11-12) are within the heart, and relate to the "I"; the lower I (9), the middle I (10), the higer I (11) and the cosmic I (the Christ conciousness) (12), where we are in the middle of the heart, the lamb (ram), the Christ conciousness.

1

When we are in the middle of the heart, we might have the imagination of standing at a cross. This cross is a little different in man, horse and dog.

In this picture I have tried to illustrate what imagination you might find in the center of the heart.

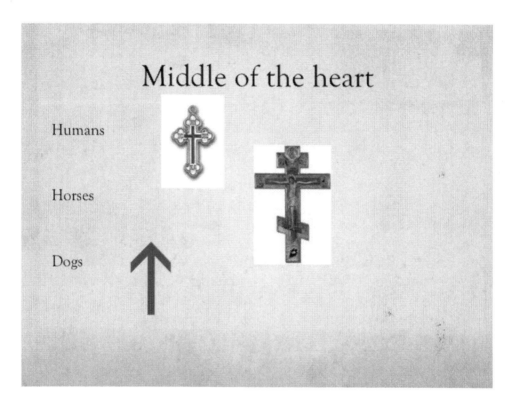

On the way through the 12 layers we may diagnose, experience and/or treat the different aspects present in these layers concerning diseases or spiritual realities.

As stated before, the two outer layers relate to the astrality of the patient; the feelings and emotions. If we stop at this layer, and take the pulse here, we get an emotional diagnosis.

- The outer layers (1-2) relate to the astral body

If we stop in the 3rd or 4th layer we will be able to diagnose the physical body. Especially interesting is the 4th layer, where we may detect the presence of parasites in the body of the patient, both physical parasites and energetic parasites.

- The 3rd - 4th layers relate to the physical body (3rd being our own physical own material body, 4th parasitic material bodies)

The layers where my students usually stop (and don't go further) are the 5th - 6th - 7th - 8th layers. Here we find the etheric forces of the body, which are the healing forces.

Most interesting is the distance between the 7th and the 8th layer. I used this distance for several years to diagnose scars of the patient, toxic scars, scars that hinder any treatment. In the 7th layer the scars were present, but in the 8th layer they were gone. So, when there was no deficiency in the 7th layer, and a clear deficiency in the 8th layer, the conclusion was that there existed a toxic scar in the process that showed deficiency in the 8th layer. I used this to **find** the scars, but I did not realize at that time that it was possible to **treat** them from the 8th ‑ 12th layer. In old days I just diagnosed them from the 8th layer, and then injected the physical scars with procaine, as described in neural therapy by Dr. Ferdinand Hünecke.

Today I know that if you go to the 8th layer or deeper (now I always go directly to the 12th layer), all forms of scar treatment is unnecessary.

- The 5th - 6th - 7th - 8th relate to the etheric body (the 4 ethers). The 7th touching the pericardium and the 8th touching the endocardium, where we leave the material world ......

The four layers within the heart itself are of immense importance. From here we may diagnose and treat diseases from the spiritual realm of the patient. This is what I think today is the right thing to do.

- The inner (9th - 10th - 11th - 12th) are within the heart, and relate to the "I"; the lower I (9th), the middle I (10th), the higher I (11th) and the cosmic I (the Christ consciousness) (12th), where we are in the middle of the heart, where the lamb (ram), the Christ consciousness resides.

When we treat from the middle of the heart, we are in the deepest spiritual realm, and there the usual stumble-stones are gone.

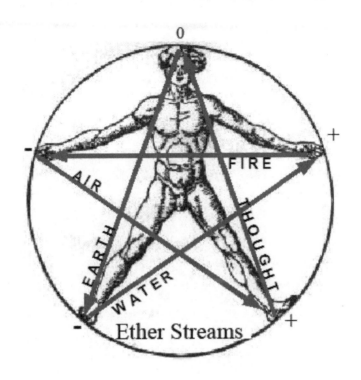

Ether Streams

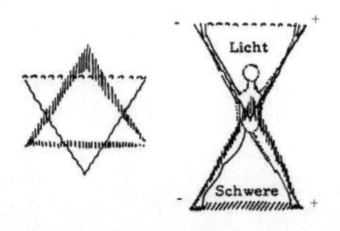

Chapter two;

A spiritual/energetic view on health and disease. The trinity contra the duality. Occidental thinking contra Oriental thinking. Luziferic, Ahrimanic and Asuric entities. Christ as the healing middle.

First, in this chapter, I will tell two personal stories that made me understand the difference between energetic and spiritual medicine.

- I had suffered from a Candida-infection in the intestines for 60 odd years, and the situation seemed impossible to solve. I had tried for several years to regulate the balance between bacteria and fungus, but it was very difficult. Then I took a "radionic nosode" of Candida (a remedy made from the frequency of the Candida fungus), and then 3 days later something interesting happened. I SAW the spirit of the Candida leave me, and in one second I was healed. Then the Candida settled in a balance with the bacteria and other microorganism, under the leadership of my own spirit, my own energetics. Then I understood how homeopathy could work against infections; it drives out the **spirit** of the microorganism, the **demon** of the disease.

- The other story happened in 1980, when I was a veterinarian in Bodø, Northern Norway. My wife at that time had a visit from a friend, and when I came into the room I SAW a "Luziferic excessive pathological structure" half way out of her left scull, half way within the head. She told me that she was suffering a painful migraine. I went towards this woman, and took hold of the energetic structure with my hand. I pulled the structure half way out, and the woman said that the pain diminished. Then I let go of the structure, and it slipped immediately back into the head of the woman. "Auuuu" she said, "now the pain has come back"! Again I grabbed hold of the Luziferic structure and pulled it all the way out. The migraine totally disappeared. This time I was very careful in what I did to the structure that I held in my hand. I went to the open window, and threw the demonic structure out. It did not return.

These two experiences became very important and influential to my life and development. They taught me that diseases are structural entities, like small living demons. However, the most important lesson did not appear to me until 20 years later; namely **where did the demonic structure go?** Did it enter another human being? Did it enter an animal? What happened to it?

Today this question has become very important to me, and is the main reason why I have written this book. When we treat patients with acupuncture or other therapies, do we just translocate the pathological structure? Do we dissolve it? How must we treat to dissolve the structure, and not just pass it on?

This book is mostly concerned with this question.
The answer is that we must treat the middle between the excess and the deficiency, with Christ-consciousness, after the principle of trinity and not duality.

In this second chapter I will further elaborate on what was said at the end of the first chapter, namely concerning the *middle.*

What importance the middle has for the disease and the healing.

Especially relating to the problem of **translocation,** which will be dealt with further in chapter three.

To be able to treat the middle, we have to understand the difference between duality and trinity. There is no middle in dualistic thinking, there is no middle between Yin and Yang.

As this could have been the subject of numerous lectures or even books, I will try to write this in a very short form.

The oriental philosophy is based on dualism, on the thinking of Yin/Yang theory. This theory has given rise to great achievements in the development of society and medicine.

In early Christian philosophy the idea of the Trinity was developed, with the;

- Three-fold God, consisting of God, Son and the Holy Spirit.
- Christ between Luzifer and Ahriman (Satan).
- Humans consisting of body-soul-spirit.
- The soul consisting of thinking, feeling and willing.

Most acupuncturists in the world treat after duality thinking, treating the excess or the deficiency. They can also balance the two with special techniques, still not treating the middle, just the balancing point.

Very few, if any, treat the middle area as such. This theory is only found in the works of Dr. Rudolf Steiner (see more about this in chapter seven).

The concept of trinity "may be" also found in the old Chinese writings.

Here follows a commentary made by **Dr. Bruce Ferguson** on my question of the existence of a trinity in the Chinese philosophy.

"Still, if one read the old books of Nei Ching, we actually do find clear indications of a trinity-thinking. Most people only think in the TCM duality, and don't consider the Trinity (and beyond). So, everyone knows about Yin and Yang, but what do they think about, for example, the San Jiao (Triple Burner)? Or even more importantly in Daoist medical theory, the 3 treasures; Qi, Jing and Shen?
Most of the diagnostic explanatory power and subsequent treatment principles in current TCM is derived from the basic duality of Yin and Yang. The Chinese character for Yin is

derived from a glyph which represents the dark cloud-shrouded side of a hill. Since that initial representation, the meaning of the word Yin has grown to include Dark, Cool, Moist, Quiet, Restive, Female, and Structure. It also, perhaps, includes more modern concepts such as omega-3 fatty acids, hypotension, vasodilation, anti-inflammatory cytokines, T-suppressor cells, and so on.

In contradistinction, the Chinese character for Yang is derived from the glyph for the sunlit side of a hill. Since then, the word Yang has expanded it's meaning to include Light, Warm, Dry, Noisy, Active, Male, South, and Function. Some more modern additions to the concept of Yang might include omega-9 fatty acids, hypertension, vasoconstriction, T-helper cells, inflammatory cytokines, and other similar biological activities and processes.

At this point it should be emphasized that the words Yin and Yang are adjectives, and not nouns. So, for example, our Sun in this solar system is Yang (hotter) compared to a cooler red-giant star, but is Yin (cooler) compared to a very hot white dwarf star. So the Sun is neither Yin nor Yang in the nominative sense, but can be considered to have Yin or Yang qualities when viewed comparatively. And a relatively active Great Dane dog (Deutsche Dogge) may be considered Yang compared to a normal Bull Mastiff, but certainly Yin in it's activity level compared to the average Jack Russel Terrier.

TCM is, at it's heart, a heteropathic medicine. After a diagnosis is made, the treatment principle opposite to the diagnosis is applied in order to bring the organism into balance. So a febrile patient (relatively Yang with respect to it's normal resting status) is given a Yin treatment (e.g. cooling herbs, foods, acupuncture treatment, etc.) in order to normalize or harmonize the patient. And, although a simple Yin and Yang designation is not usually considered a complete diagnosis, a derivation of that Duality such as the Eight Principles is commonly sufficient to diagnose and treat most disharmonies. The Eight Principles, as a reminder, is a derivation of Yin (Cool, Internal, and Deficient) and Yang (warm, external, and excess).

For example, an older canine patient with loose stools,

generalized weakness, shortness of breath, a deep, weak pulse (especially in the Cubit or middle position), mild to moderate muscle mass loss, and mildly cool, is said to have a Deficiency of Spleen Qi and the TCM heteropathic treatment principle is to Tonify Spleen Qi.

But there is more to TCM than this Yin and Yang Duality. The Daoists considered that "from the one, came the two, from the two came the three, and from the three came the ten thousand things". So, rather than a continuous arithmetic permutation of Yin and Yang leading to four (Yang within Yang, Yin within Yang, Yin within Yin and Yang within Yin, as well as the Four Seasons, and the Four Cardinal Directions) then eight (e.g. the Ba Gua, the eight trigrams, as well as the Eight Principles as noted above), then 64 (e.g. the 64 hexagrams of the I Ching), in the Daoist Trinity there is a type of creative "explosion" after three. But please note here that even the Ba Gua (Eight Trigrams) is composed of TRIGRAMS, the first hint that Duality is at least partially composed of Trinities.

Moreover, the basic principles of TCM already include notions of a Trinity in the concepts of the San Jiao (Triple Burner) and the 3 Treasures (Qi, Jing, Shen). Further, the San Jiao is not only one of the 12 basic "organs" in TCM, but San Jiao is also a specialized diagnostic system.

This Trinity is sometimes expanded into the Wu Xing or 5 Phases (mistakenly termed the "5 Elements" in the western world, a curious admixture of Chinese and Greek concepts). The Wu Xing is obviously NOT a derivation of Duality, but rather an expansion of the Daoist Trinity.

Further, in the treatment of musculoskeletal or musculotendinous pain, a commonly taught treatment strategy is the 3-needle strategy of Distal, Local, and Proximal channel points. And for Zang-Fu Organ disharmonies, a commonly employed treatment strategy is another 3-needle treatment technique of Back Shu, Front Mu, and Source point (Shu-association, Mu-alarm, and Yuan-source). So we see that the use of three or a Trinity of points for treatment in TCM is very common.

Also we must think about the 3 pulse positions and the 3 needle depths, heaven, human and earth"

When I first realized that treatment of either the excess or the deficiency caused/could cause the pathological structure to translocate, I started to search for a way that was safe to use.

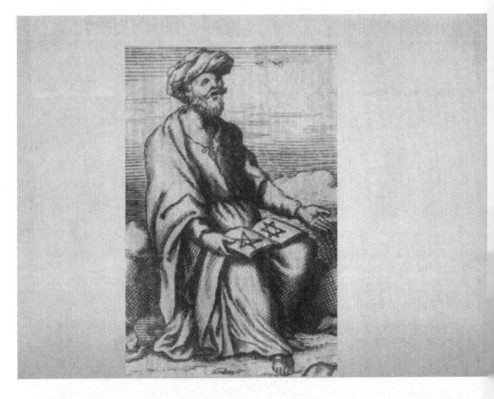

Me considering what system to use; the 5-star or the 6-star.

Dualism contra Trinity

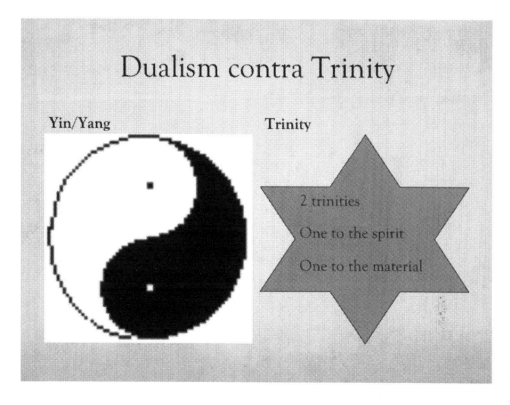

Yin/Yang   **Trinity**

2 trinities

One to the spirit

One to the material

The duality contra the trinity.

The first hint or advice I received on this matter, came from **Judith von Halle**, a woman with cosmic consciousness, who received the stigmata in 2004, living in Berlin / Dornach (Switzerland).

She told me that to avoid translocating the disease one had to treat with *"Christ consciousness"*.

What is meant by *"Christ consciousness"*?

It took me some months to understand that "Christ consciousness" was all about staying in the middle, in the middle between the excess and the deficiency, between Luzifer and the Devil (Ahriman).

Christ, even in his last minutes inside the human body of Jesus, hung in the middle between two robbers; one representing the Luziferic, the other the Ahrimanic.

The first time I tried to treat the middle, and only the middle, I was standing beside a horse together with Dr. Markus Steiner, a German college. Suddenly I SAW, quite clearly, the Ahrimanic pathological structure (in the area of the stomach of the horse) and the Luziferic pathological structure (in the area of the chest). With a violent shot from a "dermojet" I then treated the exact middle between the two, and immediately they pulled back. Accordingly to Dr. Steiner the alien entities did not leave the body entirely, but stayed in the legs. Later I found out that if I treated the middle too violently the demons did not totally go away. The middle had to be treated more with care, with a needle, or with the fingers.

Since then I have treated many human and veterinary patients following this method, using one needle carefully placed in the middle. Most of them are very satisfied with the great effect of this treatment. They describe strong energies changing and streaming through the body.

Later I have seen that the middle point is a little closer to the excess, as shown in the picture on the next page (33).

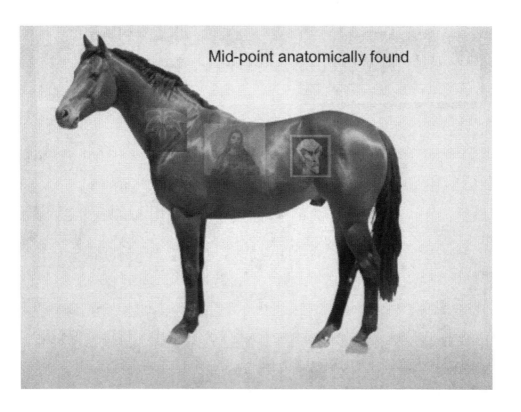
Mid-point anatomically found

The Luziferic structures are almost always proximal or cranial. The Ahrimanic structures are almost always distal or caudal.

Now, there is also another group of pathological structures, in ancient tradition called the Asuric demons. They seem not to be in connection with the Luziferic and the Ahrimanic demons, which usually balance each other. I seldom find or see these demons, so there is not much I can say about them.

- Traditionally the Luziferic demons relate to the feelings, the astral forces of the body.

- Traditionally the Ahrimanic demons relate to the growth forces of the body, the etheric forces of the body.

- Traditionally the Asuric demons relate to the spirit, the consciousness, the "I" forces of the body.

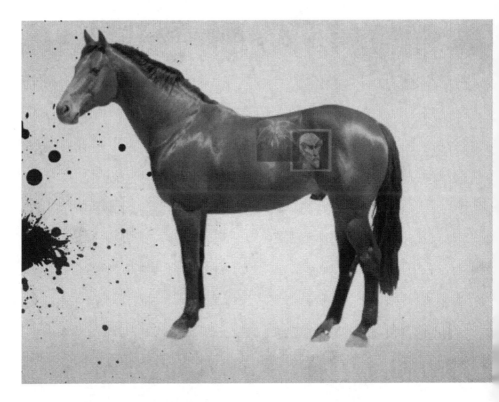

The relation between the Luziferic and the Ahrimanic demons in cancer and/or destructive energy

Chapter three;

Treating the excess. The problem of pathological translocation. Treating the pathological information.

As already spoken of, the treatment of the excess, the symptoms, will always lead to the translocation of the pathological excessive structure, the Luziferic structure, the Luziferic demon.

The deficient Ahrimanic demon is usually not addressed or touched.

The Asuric demon, if it is present, also is not addressed.

Most acupuncturists, doctors, veterinarians and physiotherapists treat the excessive structure, which manifest as symptoms.

Also many homeopaths, herbalists and even Anthroposophic doctors treat the symptoms, and through this induce a translocation of the cause of the symptoms.

This is not good.

As we all know what treatment of the symptoms means, I will not let this chapter get bigger than this.

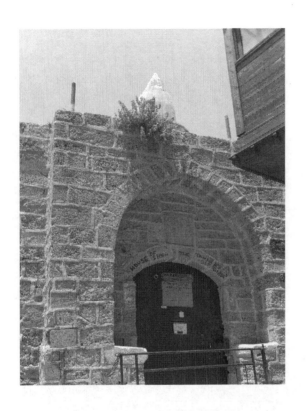

"When I visited Jaffa in Israel, I found the house where Peter visited Simon, and healed (woke up from the dead) the woman Tabitha. As I sat there outside the house, I was suddenly transported back in time and saw clearly how Peter did this. He approached the sick/dead woman and passed her (turning his back on her). Then he turned around and watched how Luzifer and Ahriman had joined together in her death, situated in her heart region. He then pressed his finger in the tiny gap between them (they can never join totally), pressed them apart, and brought Tabitha back to life".

Chapter four;

Treating the deficiency. The problem of duality. The trinity-solution. Cancer treatment.

First I will give a short description of my "old" cancer treatment when it was based on treating the deficiency (and not the middle point).

From a holistic viewpoint one evaluates the processes that control a cancerous tumor to be totally normal, even healthy. The normal biological activity is for a cell to grow and multiply. For many animals and plants this process continues throughout life. It is only in the case of highly developed animals that growth and cell division stop at a certain age. It is likewise in these species that cancer becomes a "normal" illness. If growth processes continue throughout life, cancer (uncontrolled processes) occurs to a much smaller degree. The controlling processes begin to play a more active role when growth is about to stop. They impede physical development. These controlling processes are, to an increasing degree, present the more developed the individual is; they reach their maximum in mammals. If these controlling processes fail in their function, growth processes regain dominance and cancerous tumors can arise.

Many reasons explain the failure of the controlling processes. Day after day, the processes that control all cellular and bodily functions are stressed constantly. The stressors include shock, strain on the psyche, bombardment with unwanted sounds, visual impressions, food additives and electromagnetic influences (high voltage cables, geo-phatic stress, etc.). These stressors can lead to strain on, or loss of dominance of, the controlling processes, and especially the immune system.

The aim of all cancer therapy must be to help the patient to regain this dominance and restore control of the processes, especially of the immune system, which is critical for good health. Time after time many methods, from meditation to more or less vegetarian diets, have been developed to re-establish control.

In holistic medicine it is most important to stimulate the body's controlling processes. The idea is to "bring control" to the growth processes; otherwise they become uncontrolled, which is the basic problem with cancerous cells. If we stimulate the wrong processes, we may aggravate the disorder by stimulating tumor growth. In my opinion, working via the Ko-Cycle (controlling) cycle is the best way to stimulate the controlling Processes of the body.

Treatment of patients suffering from cancer
First, we must make a meridian Diagnosis, either via pulse diagnosis (then we have to go back in time, as the cancer development started in the past), or by a simple observation of where the tumor has arisen.

When the patient suffers from cancer, it is very important to decide the location of the lesion. This will indicate the process that lost its control at the time the cancer started.

Let us take mammary cancer as an example. It manifests on the stomach (ST)-meridian (mamma is situated on the stomach-meridian). We must then particularly avoid stimulating ST-process, but we should stimulate the liver (LV), the controlling process of ST (the father of ST). For this, we could use the Ting (Wood) Point (LV01), or Earth Point (LV03) or the related ECIWO-point on the liver meridian where it passes the metatarsal bone. We should stimulate only the controlling process, not the Ko (Controlling) Point of ST itself. During the period of treatment, we should stimulate no other process, either by acupuncture, herbs, homeopathic or in any other way. However, we may combine other therapies that stimulate the liver.

I have tried this method over several years. Following my instructions several colleagues in the USA and Australia have tried it. The results have been very encouraging. Between 60-80% (depending on the organ or tissue of origin) of confirmed cancer cases have improved noticeably. The improvements included increased quality of life, better sleep, increased appetite (and in dogs a glossier coat). Overall 60% have been totally cured of the illness. Tumor(s) have, in such cases, vanished within six weeks. Two examples:

- *The first patient in whom I tried this method was a Dachshund. It had mammary cancer and probably lung metastases. I treated LV-ECIWO (ECIWO-point of the mamma on the LV-meridian). Within a few weeks the tumors were almost gone. Guess who was more amazed, the dog, the owner or I?!*
- *In liver tumors, we must stimulate only LU-Channel (Metal Controls Wood). This activates the body's control system for the liver, so that the body itself can bring the cancerous tumors under control. If we succeed in this, the active tumor tissue shrivels within a few days and disappears within a six weeks. If there is considerable fibrosis of the area, the fibrous tissue remains permanently, as is true for scars elsewhere.*

This was my cancer protocol for many years, and it worked very well. I had great success.

But, I saw more and more that the pathological information underlying the cancer symptom was not dissolved. It was just translocated, either within the body of the patient, or it was pushed over to other individuals, family, friends or animals.

After I began to treat the middle point this has not been seen.

I find the middle point relating to the excess and the deficiency in the following way;

Acupuncture-wise

First, through a thorough pulse analysis in the 12th layer, in the middle of the heart (see chapter one), I find the deficiency, the main deficiency in the pulse. If I find the main deficiency on the left hand (either HT, LV or KI, let us say in this example that it is LV), I must then further consider the two other pulses on this same hand. I must then search for and find the main excess on the same hand (either HT or KI, let us say in this example that it is KI). The middle point is then the remaining process, namely in this example HT.

If the main deficiency is on the right hand, the middle will then either be LU, SP or PC. This system is quite new, and it was initially worked out in cooperation with THP Corinne Dettmer and through discussions with Dr. Vet. Markus Steiner.

Finding the middle-point like this (acupuncture-wise)

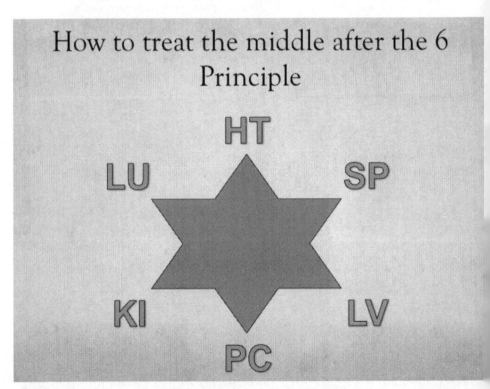

Or like this

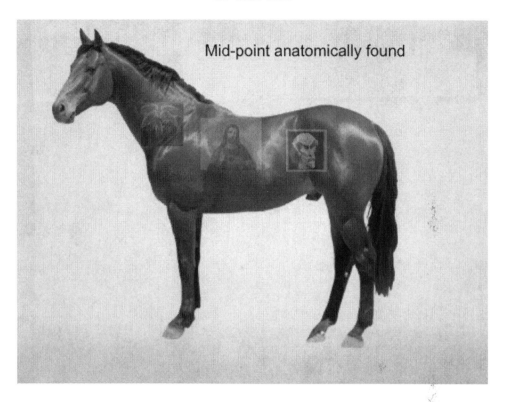

Mid-point anatomically found

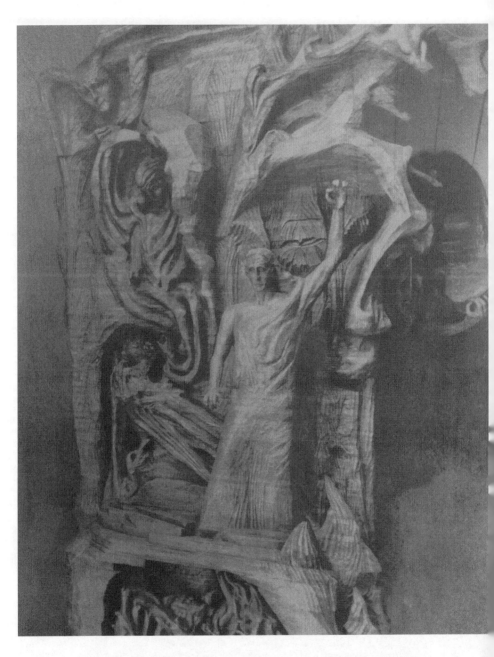

Rudolf Steiner's view of Christ, Ahriman and Luzifer

Chapter five;

Treating the middle through osteopathy and cranio-sacral work. New ways of treating cancer. The problem of evil.

Instead of finding the middle point through the 6-star as described in chapter four, and then ending up with an acupuncture meridian or point as the result, we may find the middle point anatomically, just by feeling or seeing the excess and the deficiency, or said in another way; the Luziferic and the Ahrimanic demonic structures.

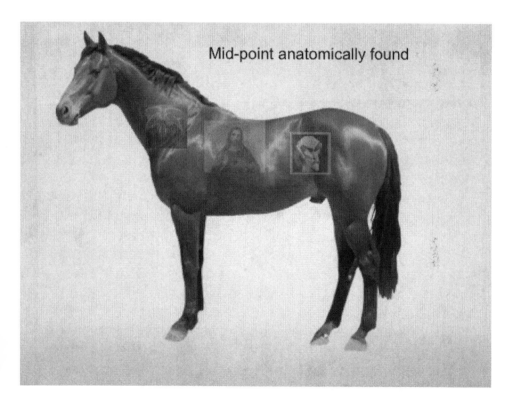

Mid-point anatomically found

The first time I SAW these demons was when I was standing beside a horse, in the company of Dr. Markus Steiner. Suddenly I saw the two demons, and then intuitively placed a shot from the dermojet in the mid-point between them. The effect was immediate. They split and pulled back. According to Dr. Markus Steiner they did not dissolve when using the dermojet, so now with all present patients, I use just a dry needle and the effect has been much better.

In the same way, when I visited Jaffa in Israel, as related earlier I found myself sitting outside the house where Peter visited Simon, and healed the woman Tabitha. He approached the sick/dead woman and passed her (turning his back on her). Then he turned around and watched how Luzifer and Ahriman had joined together in her death, situated in her heart region. He then pressed his finger in the tiny gap between them (they can never join totally), pressed them apart, and brought Tabitha back to life. This is how we might do the treatment in osteopathy or cranial-sacral therapy.

One very good example on treating the anatomical or acupuncture midpoint instead of the deficient point concerns a horse that was treated during a course at Worpswede in Germany, at the place owned by Sandra Reichelt. This horse had several problems, mainly with her behavior. We found the deficiency through Cranial-Sacral investigation as described in this book. Practically the method is to feel every point on the head with the fingers, and when the maximal excess and the maximal deficiency is found, the middle point between the two is treated, still only with the fingers. In this case the deficiency was found on the top of the head. The excess was just over the eye. The midpoint was in the middle of Os frontale. One of the students held her finger at the midpoint, and after entering into the spiritual world (as described under pulse-diagnosis), and lowering her energy into her feet, she started the therapy. Very soon the horse relaxed, and seemed to be cured. The deficiency and the excess were gone. We all stood back for a moment, looking at the horse. Then something came out of the horse, and swirled around. I felt like fainting. Some felt like drunk. It was a demon, or one might say a soul-fragment from the former owner. It went around in the circle, and showed anger for being driven out. After some minutes the demon that came out of the horse was transformed into light and disappeared. This all happened through treating the midpoint, the

44

Christ-point. Why the treatment was somewhat altered or disturbed this time, was probably because we all stood in a circle around the horse, so that the pathological energy, the pato-structure or the "demon" was sort of trapped. Then we all had to give light to release it. For me this has never happened before.

Add; a few weeks later I received a mail from one of the course participants that a part of the pathological energy (part of the demon or part of the soul-fracture of the horse) had stuck with her. She had to get help to free herself completely. This shows that the forces we are dealing with can be dangerous.

"Hallo zusammen,
beim letzten Seminar in Worpswede hab ich leider einen Selenanteil geschluckt. Dank meiner Therapeutin hat sie es schnell bemerkt und mich bei ihr zu Hause davon befreien können. Das Wesen saß fest in meinem Herzen und hat dann erneut versucht nachts von ihr Besitz zu ergreifen. Das was da war, war definitiv nicht ohne und jetzt fragen wir uns, ob noch ein Teilnehmer Veränderungen seit dem Seminar an sich bemerkt hat, bzw. ihr auch die Möglichkeit habt, das an Euch checken zu lassen. Gern stelle ich einen Kontakt zu meiner Energetikerin her.
Außerdem sollten wir mehr an Schutz und Prevention arbeiten..
Liebe Grüße ....

In English;
Hello everyone,
at the last seminar we had in Worpswede I happened to attract a part of the Demon that was released. Thanks to my therapist who was able to diagnose this quickly, and was able to release this pathological structure at her clinic, I got away without serious damage. The entity was stuck in my heart, where it tried to stick and make a new home. After this we must ask ourselves if any of the other participants in the seminar have felt something similar. If so, it is important that they get diagnosed and treated. They may come to my therapist as she now has experience with this matter. We must work more on the subject of how to prevent such things happening in the future.
Love from ....

My comment;

If some of the organs or processes of the body are "empty", such demons may easily get a hold.

The best way to prevent this of course is to stay healthy.

If we are not healthy enough, we may protect ourselves by different techniques.

- *One technique is to imagine a fire-wall around oneself.*
- *Another is to imagine a mirror between the patient and oneself.*

Such techniques must be tested out by each individual.

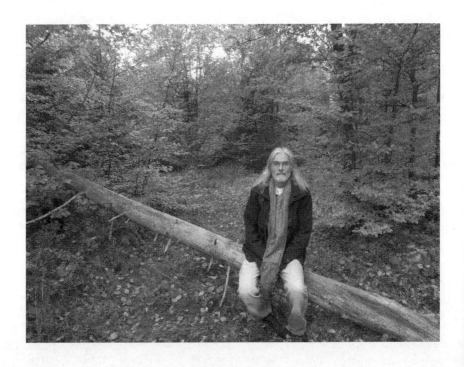

In the Norwegian woods

Chapter six;

Treating the middle through acupuncture. The 5-star versus the 6-star. A new system of acupuncture pointing towards the future.

The "old" way to treat the deficiency was directly, according to the 5-star rule.

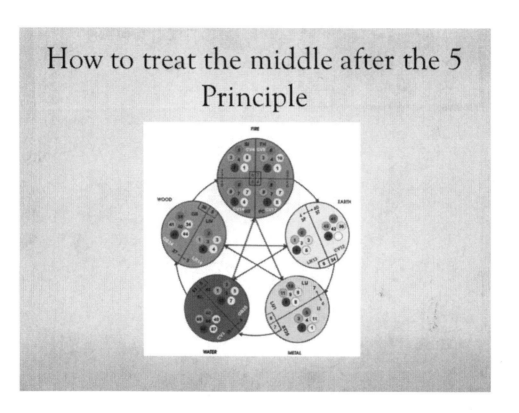

In this system the theory is as follows; let us say that we have eaten too much processed food, sugar and toxins so that the liver is weakened. Then the livers control over the next element (Earth – Spleen and Stomach) in the Ko-cyclus is weakened, and the stomach becomes excessive. Then there will then be pain, over-activity or possibly even cancer in the stomach or along the stomach meridian. The excess of the stomach will drain the spleen, and after a while the spleen will suffer deficiency. The spleen will then loose control over the water element, and the first organ (process) in the water element that will become excessive is the bladder. Then we get symptoms like bladder infection, bladder pain or bladder cancer. The excess of the bladder will then drain the kidney, which after a while become deficient. The kidneys will then loose their control over the fire element, with its four organs; the heart, the pericardium, the small intestine and the trippel burner. The two yang processes will first show the excess, namely small intestine and the trippel burner. The excessive symptoms will then appear there, giving rise to infections, pain and in the end cancer. The fire Yang processes will then drain the Yin fire processes or organs, and the heart and pericardium will be weakened, they become deficient.

And so it continues.

As earlier described there are three ways of treating this problem.

- We may treat the excess where we find it.
- We may treat the deficiency.
    - The initial or first deficiency.
    - The present deficiency.
- We may treat the middle point.
    - According to the 6-star.
    - According to the anatomical midpoint on the body.
    - According to the middle point at the scull.

Effectively to treat the excess or the deficiency we have good use of the 5-star. To treat the middle point though, we need another set-up of the different organs/processes.

This other set-up is pictured on page 40. It is the 6-star method explained in chapter 4.

As this is a new system, time will show if it must be improved or if it can stand firmly on its own ground.

Chapter seven;

Treating the onset of the disease in time. The midline. Treating the onset of the disease through the generations. Trans-generational medicine.

I have used this picture in my lectures for several years. It shows how we can go back in time with our pulses.

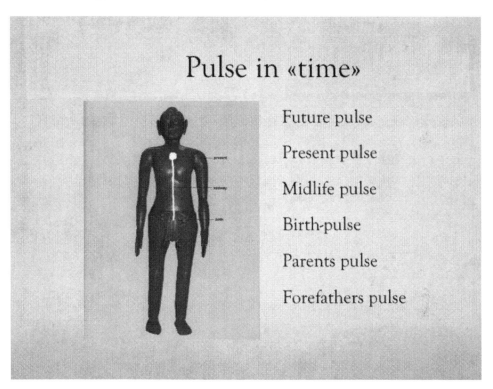

Pulse in «time»

Future pulse

Present pulse

Midlife pulse

Birth-pulse

Parents pulse

Forefathers pulse

The method is as follows;
We take the pulse, enter into the spiritual world, concentrate on our own heart and then enter into the heart of the patient all the way to the 12th layer where we are at the deepest present pulse. There we find the most deficient pulse. Holding this deficient pulse, we then start to go distal, along the midline. If the deficient pulse disappears,

let us say midway to Os pubis, the problem, the deficiency, the disease, started midway in life.

The total pulse-picture will change radically when in our mind we travel along the midline distal, which is going back in time. The distance between the center of the heart and Os pubis resembles the total life span. Midway resembles midway in life. Os pubis resembles the birth, and so on. We just have to follow the main deficient pulse all the way through life, to find the onset of the problem. Sometimes it goes right the way to birth, all the way to Os pubis, and sometimes beyond. What does this imply?

Now, one of my students, Margit Buen, a nurse who works with trans-generational trauma, found that we can continue below the Os pubis. We can continue down the legs. The father line is in the left leg, and the mother line is in the right leg. The total life span of the parents is in the length of the thigh, Os femur, and in the knee junction we find the birth of the parents. Then in Os tibia we find the life of the grandfathers, and in Os fibula the life of the grandmothers. In the Os tarsales we find the great-grand mothers and fathers. It seems that we can follow the forefathers- and mothers through 7 generations.

The treatment of this pre-generational onset of disease through different forms of trauma (like war, prison, concentration camps, rape, murder and so on) is to put a needle, with intent and knowledge, exactly at the point of the onset of the disease, at the starting point of the deficiency.

calcaneus
  talus
cuboid
navicular
cuneiform

ADDENDUM I;

Pulse diagnosis as an initiation to the spiritual world

Rudolf Steiner describes the foundation for developing the necessary state of mind like this;

"Between birth and death man, at his present evolutionary stage, lives in ordinary life through three soul states: waking, sleeping, and the state between them, dreaming. Man acquires knowledge of higher worlds if he develops consciousness during sleeping. During its waking state the soul surrenders itself to sense-impressions and thoughts that are aroused by these impressions. During sleep the sense-impressions cease, but the soul also loses its consciousness. The experiences of the day sink into the sea of unconsciousness. Let us now imagine that the soul might be able during sleep to become conscious despite the exclusion of all sense-impressions. An answer to this problem is only possible if the soul is able to experience something even though no sense-activities and no memory of them are present in it. The soul, in regard to the ordinary outer world, would then find itself in a state similar to sleep, and yet it would not be asleep, but, as in the waking state, it would confront a real world. Such a state of consciousness can be induced if the human being can bring about the soul experiences made possible by spiritual science; and everything that this science describes concerning the worlds that lie beyond the senses.

This state of consciousness resembles sleep only in a certain respect, namely, through the fact that all outer sense-activities cease with its appearance; also all thoughts are stilled that have been aroused through these sense-activities. Through it a perceptive faculty is awakened in the soul that in ordinary life is only aroused by the activities of the senses. The soul's awakening to such a higher state of consciousness may be called initiation.

The means of initiation lead from the ordinary state of waking consciousness into a soul activity, through which spiritual organs of observation are employed. These organs are present in the soul in a germinal state; they must be developed. It may happen that a human being at a certain moment in the course of his life, without special preparation, makes the discovery in his soul that such higher organs have developed in him. This has come about as a sort of involuntary self-awakening. Such a human being will find that through it his entire nature is transformed. A boundless enrichment of his soul experiences occurs. He will find that there is no knowledge of the sense world that gives him such bliss, such soul satisfaction, and such inner warmth as he now experiences through the revelation of knowledge inaccessible to the physical eye. Strength and certainty of life will pour into his will from a spiritual world. — There are such cases of self-initiation. They should, however, not tempt us to believe that this is the one and only way, and that we should wait for such self-initiation, doing nothing to bring about initiation through proper training. How the human being may develop through training the organs of perception that lie embryonically in the soul will be described here."

By combining the three qualities (not caring, not mind-wandering and not acting) one concentrates on the patient but does not interfere with his/her energies. Done in this way, diagnostic pulse taking is as detached and objective as possible.

Our mind may very well influence the result in our diagnostic work, just in the same way that the observer may influence the outcome in quantum physics.
When we try to take the pulse, we should also be as relaxed as possible, without muscular tension.   *colleagues*
We should also avoid the presence of critical observers, colleges who are aggressive about what we do or competitors who are jealous of our good results.

52

What I have observed in connection to my pulse-taking, is the same as what is described in the book "The secret life of plants" by **Peter Tompkins** and **Christopher Bird.** They describe that we have to be in a meditative state of mind for the plants to be able to "sense" human feelings, the feelings of man. This book describes how it is possible for us to get into emotional contact with plants, and how the presence of jealous or aggressive persons completely diminished the contact described.

This contact is very similar to what we must obtain with the patient or animal in pulse-taking.

This same conclusion was made by the French scientist **Beneviste** in his investigations on homeopathy. Homeopathy seems not to work when we are not meditatively tuned into the remedy when it is made, or when it is given out to the patient.

Hahnemann described the same phenomenon in his "Organon der Heilkunst", 6th edition, § 265.

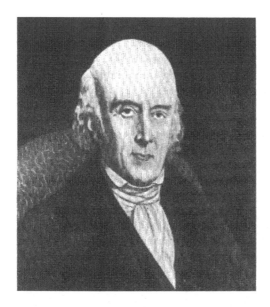

Christian Frederic Samuel Hahnemann

§. 265.

Es ist Gewissenssache für ihn, in jedem Falle untrüglich überzeugt zu seyn, daß der Kranke jederzeit die rechte Arznei einnehme, *und deßhalb muß er die \ richtig -/ gewählte Arznei \ dem Kranken/ ⸗ aus seinen eignen Händen \ [1271] / geben, auch sie selbst[1272] ⸗zubereiten[1273] I).[1274]*

[1275] *I) Um dieses wichtige Grundprincip meiner Lehre aufrecht zu erhalten, habe ich seit dem Beginne ihrer Entdeckung viele Verfolgungen erduldet.*

#

Today I would describe the way of entering the spiritual world as follows;

The main "thing" or constellation or configuration that hold us with a fast grip in the physical world is the entanglement of Thinking, Feeling and Willing. As long as we are in this grip we will not be able to detect the energetic changes in the spiritual world. We have then to separate Feeling from Willing and Thinking in order to enter the "other-world".
All past esoterics or shamans have been faced with this problem, and they have developed methods in how to enter the spiritual world. When not using drugs or plants these methods are quite similar to what I have here described; separating either the

dimensions of the world (depth – width – height – time), or the faculties of the soul (willing – feeling – thinking).

It is interesting to note that the modern "Elf-school" in Iceland uses much the same method.

There is a close connection between the directions in this physical world, and the three soul-qualities of Thinking, Feeling and Willing. Thinking is directed upwards (Cosmos), Feeling to the periphery (the wide expanses of the world), and Willing is directed downwards, to the earth itself. If we then let ourselves fade out into the wide expanses of the world, as we do when meeting a situation that does not interest us, and we almost fall asleep.

#

The pulse diagnosis as a way to clairvoyant observation, described in connection with the anthroposophy of Rudolf Steiner.

Rudolf Steiner's anthroposophy describes a way to obtain spiritual knowledge. This way consists of;

- Preparation
- Imagination
- Inspiration
- Intuition

In many of his lectures and books Steiner describes how this way may be followed or walked.

After using pulse diagnosis for 29 years I realized in 2009 that the spiritual development I had experienced through developing my skills within pulse diagnosis, had clear and distinct parallels to Steiner's description of the path that a spiritual disciple has to walk.

First a short résumé of my development in pulse diagnosis.

In the beginning the pulse observations were very fragile; I had to be newly washed, in quiet surroundings, neither hungry or full; in short I needed to be in a balanced state of mind. After some years this became less and less important as the observations became more and more stable. Additionally, after some years I began to literally **see** the etheric energy that I first detected through the pulse. Working with the energies of the body gave rise to the development of spiritual sense organs. First I saw the etheric energy in and between trees, then in animals and then in humans. First the observations had its sensory center in the back of the brain, but then it started to wander. First it wandered towards the heart, then the spine, and then slowly spread out through the entire body. The observations also became enlarged from an intellectual observation to an immediate knowledge of past, present and future of the puls observation. The direction of the observation, which now had become knowledge, also changed. In the beginning the direction of the information streamed from the surroundings or the patient towards me, but then it started to go both ways, as if the patient also received treatment at the same time as I was diagnosing. The observation also enlarged in space, as it came to include also the astral part. This part was seen as a light flowing area, together with the darker etheric energy.

Then the observation started to move in time. Past, present and future became one.

When I found Steiner's description of the development of Inspiration, for example in "Geisteswissenschaft im Umriss" around the pages 225 and 226, I found this to be an accurate description of what I had experienced during the last 29 years. Although Steiner's description starts with the development in the astral body, which then spreads to the etheric body, the development connected to the pulse seems to start in the etheric body spreading to the astral body.

#

In a lecture held on August 26, 1912 in Munich, Rudolf Steiner also describes how important the hands are as spiritual sense-organs, and by this he predicts the importance of the pulse diagnosis, where **the sensitive fingertips meet the consciousness of the blood stream**;

"…. that is what we experience when we try to find the relation between that part of the human or etheric body, which corresponds to the brain or head, and the physical brain or physical head itself. There is an intimate connection between them. If we want to express the relation, we may say that in our head, especially in our brain, we have a faithful expression of the etheric forces, something that, in the external phenomena and external functions, gives us a really faithful image of the functions and processes in the corresponding etheric part.

It is different in the case of other organs of the human etheric body and the corresponding physical sense organs. **Consider the hands**. The difference between the external physical hands and their tasks, and what lies at the basis of the corresponding etheric part is far greater than the difference between the physical head and its corresponding part in the human etheric body. What is done by the etheric organ called the hands does manifest only in a small degree in what finds physical expression in the hands. The etheric organs of the hands are true spiritual organs. The etheric organs expressed in the hands and their functions, work far more intuitively, more spiritually, and perform a far higher task than is accomplished by the etheric brain. Whoever has made progress in these matters will say that the brain with its etheric basis is in effect by far the least skillful of the spiritual organs man bears within him.

*The spiritual activities connected with the organs underlying the hands, but incompletely expressed in the hands and their functions, serve a far higher, more spiritual kind of knowledge and observation. **These organs can lead into the super-sensible world and can occupy themselves with our perception and orientation there**. A spiritual seer may express this, somewhat surprisingly but accurately, by saying that the human brain is a most clumsy organ for research in the spiritual world, and that the hands, or the spiritual basis of the hands, are far more interesting and significant organs for gaining knowledge of the world, and are certainly far more skillful organs than the brain.*

Not much is gained on the way to initiation by advancing from the use of the physical brain to a free use of the etheric brain. The difference is not great between what may be achieved through a purified, intuitive brain-thinking, and regulated spiritual working in the etheric spiritual counterpart of the brain. The difference is much greater between what our hands accomplish in the world, and what can be done by the etheric part that is the spiritual basis of the hands, than the etheric brain can do as the spiritual basis of the physical brain. On the path of initiation not much development of the etheric brain is necessary, since it is not a particularly important organ. But the etheric basis of the hands is connected with the activity of the lotus flower in the region of the heart, as you will learn in my book; "Knowledge of the Higher Worlds and Its Attainment".

This lotus flower pours out its rays of force in such a way as to build up the organism that, at the stage at which physical man now stands, exists in an incomplete form in the hands and their functions. Though it may sound strange, yet it is true that the least skillful organ for spiritual investigation is the brain, since it is the least capable of development. On the other hand, entirely new perspectives are opened out when we consider other apparently subordinate organs."

Rudolf Steiner's 7 Class-lectures[4] held in Dornach as a road prescription for both therapy and for the road to Initiation.

The 19 lessons of the Michael School may reveal a path for every man and woman, as long as we read or contemplate them on a personal level. It was actually Rudolf Steiner's wish that we did not just quote these lessons, but internalized them and reshaped them from a personal experience of the spiritual.

After reading Rudolf Steiner's 7 "Recapitulation Class Lessons", that were given in Dornach between 6. and 20. September 1924, and then contemplating them as a personal instruction from the "Guardian of the Threshold" in how to penetrate into the spiritual realm of the therapeutic field, I have found so much help and clarity shining onto my path that I want to share some of this light with my colleges in the medical field.

I will show how the description of the path of initiation in these lectures almost exactly correspond to my own lifelong attempts to delve into my patients etheric and astral forces by spiritual means, mediated through the pulse-diagnosis. How these lessons can give assurance that we are on the right path, and also give the necessary corrections of the individual path or suggestions of beneficial or needed corrections.

When we set forth on such a task, we need to read all the 7 lectures one after the other in a single stream, with the intention of understanding the medical way and the path of the doctor in mind.

---

[4] *Der Meditationsweg der Michaelschule, Ergänzungsband, Die Wiederholungsstunden, Perseus Verlag, Basel, ISBN 978-3-907564-87-5*

Then we will see a therapeutic path starting to reveal itself before our eyes.

I will write this in three ways;

- First I will describe how I perform my therapy.
- Then I will describe the 7 lessons in a systematical way relating to my way of therapy.
- Then the 7 lessons will be described in a phenomenological way, still relating to my way of therapy.

Phenomenological description on diagnosis and therapy

When I meet a patient, I first;

1. See the patient, in the physical world, all the features of the person. Also I ask for the physical symptoms.
2. Then I leave the physical patient by going into the distance. I separate feeling from thinking and willing. By this separation of feeling from thinking and willing, I am capable of entering the spiritual world
3. When I enter the spiritual world it feels that my surroundings get somewhat darkened. In the physical world I also take leave of thinking and willing.
4. In entering the spiritual world, I have to take leave of my own ego-centered feeling, and enter a sort of cosmic feeling. Later, when I consider the diagnosis (thinking) and treat (willing) I also have to leave my own thinking and willing, and try to use only the divine, cosmic thinking and willing.
5. Then, I enter the diagnostic process, going through the 12 layers into the heart. The 9th layer represented by the endocard where we leave the physical. From there I have to "push" (use willing strength) to get into the spiritual. At the 12th layer we find a cross (Christ). The shape of the cross in the middle of the heart is somewhat different between

animals and humans. In humans I find a plain protestantic cross. In horses I find a Russian orthodox cross, and in the dogs I find an arrow like cross.

6. After going through the 12 layers of the patient, I have to choose the appropriate system to use in my treatment; the system of 2, 3, 4, 5, 7 or 12.

7. Then we come to the mystery of "The turning around", re-entering the physical realm for the first time, going back from the spiritual. Re-entering the physical is necessary to see if the decisions I have made concerning the therapy will be fruitful and right. Here I often feel sadness for the patient, in seeing that effect of the disease, the Karma of the disease. Here I mingle all ways of therapy to see in imaginations which one is the best.

8. Then the finding of the middle, Christ, the Controlling process. ... then I must let the will of the Gods come forth ....

9. And then I treat or stimulate the middle in addition to the more specific therapy. This is the second turning around....

Systematical description on the 7 lessons

In the first lesson the material world is described, in all it's glory, but without any possibility to find the true meaning of our existence, or our diseases; the spiritual foundation of the disease must be found elsewhere. Here we find the first and most fundamental command, without which we can´t proceed. We must keep our heart open. We must also feel the longing for the spirit, together with the adoration of the creation. Then, with an open heart, and open spiritual ears, with a longing for the spirit and an adoration for the creation, we must pass the abyss to the spiritual world, to find the true cause of the disease. The next thing we must do is to send our gaze, our eyes, out into the distance. This is also the first thing I do when I am about to examine a patient. I have to let my soul, my consciousness, my gaze, fade out into the distant areas of the creation. By doing this, I start the separation of my feeling from the thinking (which is above) and my willing (which is below). To pass the abyss we need to acquaint ourselves with the three forces of our soul; the thinking, the feeling and the willing. To do so we must separate them to a certain extent. I do this when I approach a patient, I try to become totally aware of these three soul forces, and how I can differentiate them from one another, both in myself as well as in the patient. Already 30 years ago I felt a darkness around me when I did this, and this is also described in the first lesson; we approach a dark, night-like wall, and this wall is the beginning of a deep darkness, the spiritual world, into which we are about to enter. In this darkness we can and must hear with the heart, and this hearing with the heart is the only door to knowledge. Just behind the darkness, in front of the abyss that separates us from the spiritual world, we meet the Guardian of the threshold, and he make us aware of the difficulties we may meet while we separate the three soul forces; in our thinking we meet the hatred, which must be met by love, in the feeling we meet the doubt, which must be met with hope, and in our willing we meet the fear, which must be met by courage.

In the second lesson (and also at the end of the first) it is described how we must be aware of the faults and wrongs, the mistakes and shortcomings in out feelings, our thoughts and in our will. This is described as three animals. We have to become aware of out thinking, which is dead. We have to see our feeling, which is half dead and half unconscious, and we should be aware of our willing, which is powerful and alive, but still totally unconscious. When I meet the patient I have always used a very old method to enter the spiritual by separating the three soul powers, and become aware of them and their weaknesses.

The key to this method we find described in **the third lesson**, where the directions of the three soul powers are described; the thinking above, the feeling in the far reaches of the surroundings, and the will beneath. I consciously fade into the surroundings, leaving the thoughts and will behind, delving into the feeling. Then my physical world gets darker, I am unable to think and my will is gone, I am totally in the feeling. In this state I am free of the laws of the physical world, and can travel outside my body. In this state I feel the warmth of the feeling, the light of the thinking and the life of the willing, as further described in the third lesson. The first time I returned from the spiritual world I experienced the utmost despair upon realizing that my thoughts were dead and dark, my feelings were dead and cold and my will was dead and full of death. With this first-time experience in the back of my head, this option (death of the soul) is always present, always a possibility, and I see the animals each time I diagnose in this way. Then, being in the vast distance of the surroundings, I create a tunnel between my own heart and the heart of the patient, and enter the patient's heart. It is very difficult to enter totally at the heart, so the last few centimeters I have to push, push with my will.

This pushing is described in **the fourth lesson** as a necessity. The will has here to enter the feeling, and together they must push. Then I enter a sacred room, where I am in the etheric of the patient. Then I must activate my fingers, the tip of my fingers, and they must press against the body of the patient, especially at some blood vessel. Often I use Arteria radialis, but any place may be used. Then there is created a total link between my feeling heart, my etheric fingers and my thinking. Then starts the diagnostic work. I then have to consider the disease of the patient; can it be understood from a trinity?

In the fourth lesson these relations are described, almost suddenly, without a proper relation to the rest of the lesson. I experience the same in the patient. When I am inside the etheric of the patient the following questions arise; shall I consider him/her in relation to the 4 elements? Should I then consider him/her from the view of the 5 elements? What about the 7 planets that are revealed in the organs, and should I consider or evaluate the patient in relation to the 12 Zodiac Signs, revealed in the 12 meridians or the 12 processes? Every one of these possibilities are revealed in the 12 depths, in the 12 layers of the body.

- The outer layer (1-2) relate to the astral body

- The next (3rd-4th) to the material body (3rd being our own physical own material body, 4th parasitic material bodies)
- The 5th-6th-7th-8th to the etheric (the 4 ethers) body (the 7th touching the pericardium and the 8th touching the endocardium), where we leave the material world ......
- The inner (9th-10th-11th-12th) are within the heart, and relate to the "I"; the lower I (9th), the middle I (10th), the higher I (11th) and the cosmic I (the Christ consciousness) (12th), where we are in the middle of the heart, the lamb (ram), the Christ consciousness.

These relationships are indicated at the end of the 4th lesson.

In the fifth lesson we are lectured about the necessity to allow our Will to enter the Thinking, and the Thinking to enter the Will, otherwise cosmic Thinking will take us over, and we will be unable to think from our own I. Furthermore the cosmic Will will overtake us, and our Will becomes unusable. This happens also in the therapeutic process, where I let the Will and the Thinking mingle with each other, but always staying connected with the heart. It is as if the powers of the heart stream outwards, and in this process attract the will and the thinking. As such, the three soul forces then become one, and we are able to enter from the diagnostic to the therapeutic.

This is described in **the sixth (and seventh) lesson.**
The sixth lesson describes further how important it is that the thinking is supported, even connected to the will. The thoughts must be willed in an outward movement, out into the world. The Will should also be infused with the thinking, or else it will only work on its own. This fusing of Will and Thought **must** appear at the end of the diagnostic work; the impulse of the diagnosis must ascend into the therapy, into the world´s creative reality. The Feeling must be met by its own reality, by Feeling itself. When in the spiritual world we meet the patient in such a way, first as a free spirit with the Thinking-Feeling and Willing more or less separated, then as a diagnostic and lastly as a therapist, we of course face the dangers of

passing the threshold. In lesson 6 we actually cross the threshold, and then a fundamental change occurs. Thinking and Willing and Feeling part. We can then see Thinking as light. We can then see Will as dark fire. Then Thinking goes into the Will and brings the thoughts into our self. Between the Thinking light and the fiery Will, the Feeling appears. All becomes **cosmic**. Karma and heritage works in our Will. Thoughts appear simultaneously in our head and in Cosmos.

SHAU DIE DREI.
Erlebe des Kopfes weltgestalt.
Empfinde des Hertzens Weltenschlag.
Erdenken der Glieder Weltenkraft.

SEE THE THREE.
Experience the world construction of the head.
Feel the world beating of the heart.
Think the power of the world in the limbs.

We must then Will the thoughts. The thoughts become cosmic. We must let our Feeling flow outwards, one stream to Thinking and one to Willing. Then the Feeling becomes Gloria. We must Think our Will. Then the Will becomes Moral.

Then we have to be aware of the five precautions Rudolf Steiner has described elsewhere; Rudolf Steiner tells us that when we cross the threshold of the spiritual world we need to develop the 'right' moods. There are five such moods which Rudolf Steiner calls vowels.

The first is the mood or vowel pertains *to trust. When we cross the threshold we face death and in facing death we must trust in the spiritual world, that we will continue to live. This is like a feeling of being held in the lap of the gods. This is a* *feeling of powerlessness which eventually becomes selflessness.*

__The second mood or vowel__ pertains to our ability to live into everything we come across consciously, that is, metamorphosis. The vowel of metamorphosis is necessary so that we can consciously unite with everything, pour ourselves out and allow ourselves to be made full by another. This is true love.

__The third mood or vowel__ pertains to a feeling for evil. We perceive within us what has created a duality in us, we perceive evil as a part of us, we understand that it is this ability to enter into others, metamorphosis, which, when used incorrectly leads to evil. If we know how others 'tick' we can manipulate them. That is also what the adversarial powers do to us!

__The fourth mood or vowel__ pertains to a feeling for who we are, we must learn to remember ourselves so that in crossing the threshold we don't become confused with others, so we don't become what we see and bring that back with us across the threshold. This is a mood of discernment that can only come when we have understood our own evil, and faced our own death.

__The fifth mood or vowel__ pertains to a feeling for the meaning of everything. It is becoming one with the word. What this really means is that once we cross the threshold (albeit inwardly or outwardly) one has to have learnt the language, the colors, gestures, and origins of the things we see and take into us and understand them. We can follow what we see, read, hear, to the source - and know what it is.

In **the seventh lesson** the most important aspect is the turning around and looking back at the human part of ourselves, as we are in the physical world. This is precisely what I must do as a therapist, when I want to finish, or finalize, the therapeutic process. The patient, human or animal, is in the first six lessons taken apart, as am I. We are analyzed, diagnosed, treated, healed, and then everything is put together again. We return to the physical world, back into the material/physical reality. Thus we close the journey, the quest, into the therapeutic world. Before we go back into the physical/material world, we must finish the therapeutic work. We now see the animals of the Abyss, we also see the Luziferic and Ahrimanic elemental beings, or Demons as they were called in old times, and we are able to place Christ right in the middle (therapy nr. 9).

The activation of Christ in the middle between Luzifer and Ahriman create a balancing principle, and the symptoms and causes, the excesses and deficiensies are dissipated. If we are to address the cooperation of Luzifer and Ahriman, as the creators of disease in the body, we first have to show them our back, and then turn around to face them. If we approach them directly they are more easily translocated, and just driven to other parts of the body or even to other entities, humans or animals.

This is the deep mystery of the turning around. The deficiencies are balanced out and disappear completely.

Phenomenological description on the 7 lessons

Rudolf Steiner here first describes the difference between the physical world and the spiritual world relating to time. This is done in the central mantra;

"O man, know yourself"……. Because your thinking's power is lost in times destroying stream ..…".

"O Mensch, erkenne dich selbst .... weil du des Denkens kraft verlierst im Zeitvernichtungsstrome ..…".

Here we get the feeling of how we can live in both the spiritual world and the physical world, but that there are different laws relating to these two worlds.
In pulse diagnosis I go from causality, which is "shein-zeit", illusionary time, to spiritual time, real time, endless time ... what we normally call time, I will here call causality, cause and effect .... In the Spirit, the time *is* (what I call real time, before it gets corrupted by materialism and destroys the power of real spiritual thinking, thinking power. Real time *is* a continuum ..... So we go from cause /effect to continuum and then to understanding .... as described in the first and the second lesson (therapy description stage 1 and 2) .... concerning thinking; from the dead to living to understanding .... as in the animals of the abyss. Then the animals are described, we see them as a phenomenon (lesson 1). Then we need to transform the animals (lesson 2). Then we experience the living of the real thinking (red), the real feeling (yellow) and real willing (blue) (lesson 2-3)... Then the dangers in the real living are experienced, as loosing ourselves in the spiritual world (lesson 3) (therapy description stage 4). This can be counteracted if we are able to obtain the balance in Christ (3-4. lesson) (therapy description stage 5).

So, in a way the first lesson describes the animals, the second what they are and the third how they may be conquered. ....

At the last part of the third lesson the directions of the feeling, willing and thinking are described (will downwards, thinking upwards and feeling in the surroundings), and the danger in going too far in these directions (therapy description stage 2-3).

Then the three forces of the soul are described, and how they may be overwhelmed by gravitation, and how we then have to find Love and bravery not to be lost (lesson 3) (therapy description stage 4). Then more specific at the end of the third lesson how darkness may overwhelm thinking, cold overwhelm feeling and death overwhelm will (in going too far in the three directions). We then see that it is in the balancing that the right way is found, where the Christ dwells, I might say. In the 4th lesson the balance is further described, especially relating to feeling where Luzifer and Ahriman meet in warmth and cold.

When we master this balance we can start to know the 4 elements. And then we continue with the 7 planets, and 12 zodiac signs (therapy description stage 6). At this point of experiencing the world, the touch (German; "tasten") is of special importance; and to touch is the central part of pulse-diagnosis. Body is earth. Touch is water. Life is air. Feeling is fire. We feel ourselves in the elements. Then we are told that the earth is our support. That water is our creator (German; "bildner"). Then we feel that the air is our nurse (German; "pfleger"). Then we think that our etheric streams are helped by the fire. This is the prelude to the later "thinking the will" and "willing the thinking" ..... Then we must consider the 7 planets. After that we must consider the zodiac of 12. As earlier described we then must decide for the practical therapy. Then we must visualize a total division in (1-2-3-4-5-6-7-8) 9 "beams" (therapy description stage 6). The 9 light beams relate to the stage where we enter the "I" (therapy description stage 5).

In the 5th Lesson we start with recapitulation, and then for the first time the turning around is touched upon (therapy description stage 7). The first turning around, this time before the threshold, is then described. The next will be after the crossing of the threshold in lesson 6. The Guardian of the threshold say here that when we go back into the physical world we must follow the laws of the physical world, which are different from the spiritual world. When we go back we must go with our thinking in the earth element, with the feeling in the water element, with the will in the air element. Then we feel in the air element. We also feel fear for our old animal-like thinking; personally I feel sorrow (therapy description stage 7).

To avoid this we must moderate our will by thinking in the earth. Likewise the feeling must be moderated by being awake in the water. The thinking must be moderated by experiencing the will being awakened in the air.
All is mingling ...... Thinking to feeling, thinking to earth, will to air and thinking (therapy description stage 7).

What is interesting though, is that when we come back into the physical, we have to **push** to get behind the thoughts and back into the spiritual, the Spirit-world behind the physical thoughts.
Then we need understanding and compassion for human pain (for the physical world), so that we do not fall into illusion through thinking. Further we need love for the physical world so that the feeling will not fall into illusion.
The will must feel the will of the Gods in order not to be corrupted when coming back into the physical world (therapy description stage 8).

We need *faith, hope and love* to clean *will, thought and feeling*.

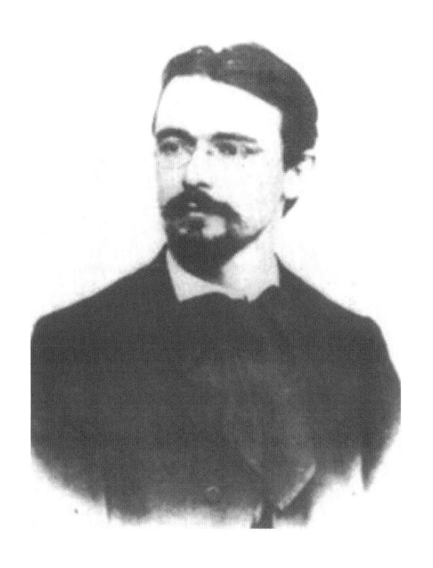

Rudolf Steiner

ADDENDUM II;

The possible use of homeopathic remedies made from the Metals, the Lanthanides and the Actinides to fight the adversaries.
A preliminary system.
This system is under development, and I will be happy to receive results or hints or advices from my honored colleges.

The Actinides work against the "atomic" power of the Asuras. They activate the healing powers against the Asuras destruction of the consciousness, and the ether of life. The symptoms are often from the "I" and/or the physical body. There are 15 actinides, just as there are about 15 main groups of Asuras entities/demons;

Aktinium	Its chemistry is dominated by (+3) O.S. Its compounds are colorless. There are 29 known isotopes. It does not have absorption in the UV visible region between 400-1000nm. ^{227}Ac is strongly radioactive and so are its decay components. Actinium metal is silvery solid; obtained by reduction of oxide, fluoride or chloride w/ Group 1 metals; and oxidized rapidly in moist air. It forms insoluble fluoride and oxalate ($Ac_2(C_2O_4)_3 \cdot 10H_2O$) compounds	Spleen
Thorium	Thorium was discovered by Berzelius in 1828 and named for the Norse god of thunder, Thor. It is a gray, radioactive metal, which is fairly abundant in the earth's crust (more than twice as much as tin) and is the first of the so-called "actinide" series, which ends with lawrencium (element 103). The long half-life of the principal isotope, Th-232, (about 1010 years) insures that there will be plenty for quite some time to come! The metal is fairly soft and malleable but darkens slowly in air due to oxidation. It reacts slowly with water at room temperature. Applications of thorium include some special magnesium alloys and photosensors. The oxide is used in high-quality lenses. An isotope of thorium can be "bred" into	Spleen

	uranium-234 by bombardment with slow neutrons. The U-234 is a fissile form of uranium and can be used in power plants.	
Protactinium	It has been in existence longer than any other actinide. ^{231}Pa has a half-life of $3.28*10^{14}$, which allows it to make chemical study easy for it. It has α-emission, so it has appropriate radiochemical precautions. The Pa metal is malleable, ductile, silvery, and has a melting point of about 1565°C. It is also a superconductor.	All Yin right sic = SP06
Uranium	Many compounds exist between the O.S. of +3 to +6. The main O.S. are +4 and +6. Stability of O.S. U^{3+} reduces to hydrogen. U^{4+} stable in aqueous solution in the absence of air. U^{5+} disproportionates rapidly into a mixture of U^{4+} and U^{6+} in aqueous solutions. U^{6+} stable in aqueous solutions. When pure it has a silvery appearance. When attacked by air, yellow film then black coating develops, it is a mix of oxide and nitride. Powder metal is pyrophoric in air. Reacts readily with hot water to prevent substances from coming into contact in nuclear reactors.	All process weak = LU01
Neptunium	It was the first transuranium element to be discovered in 1940. There are 15 known isotopes, only ^{237}Np, w/ half-life of 2.14, 10^6 years, is useful for chemical experiments. It exhibits O.S. of +3 to +7 in compounds. It is a silvery metal, with a melting point of 637°C and a boiling point of 4174°C. It has surface oxidation when exposed to air. It is converted to NpO_2 at high temperatures.	Ren mc
Plutonium	There are 15 known isotopes. The masses range from 232 to 246.The most important isotope is ^{239}Pu because it is fissionable and has a half-life of 24,100 years, which makes it easy for chemists to study. It exhibits O.S. from +3 to +7. The +3 and +4 O.S. are the most important, but compounds of the ions are well defined. Pu^{+7} only exists under very alkaline conditions. It has 6 allotropic metal forms, which makes it unusual. They can form at normal pressure between room temperature and its melting point, 640°C.It is dense, silvery and a reactive metal; more reactive than uranium or neptunium.	Kidney

	When attacked by air, it forms a green-gray oxide coating. It reacts slowly with cold water, faster with dilute H_2SO_4, and dissolves quickly in dilute hydrochloric acid or hydrobromic acid.	
Americium	It has 12 known isotopes. Americum was first made in 1944-1945 by Seaborg and his coworkers, when they decayed ^{239}Pu and ^{241}Pu to ^{241}Am, which has a half-life of 433 years, ^{241}Am and ^{243}Am, which has a half-life of 7380 years, are the most important isotopes, because their half-lives allow scientists to study their characteristics. The metal is a slivery, ductile and very malleable. It tarnishes in air slowly and dissolves in dilute hydrochloric acid quickly. It reacts with heating with oxygen, halogens, and other nonmetals	Lung
Curium	**Later Actinides (Cm, Bk, Cf, Es, Fm, Md, No, and Lr)** Their chemistry is of mostly the M^{+3} state. They all form binary compounds, such as trihalides. Curium, berkelium, and californium have the following chemistry: Oxidized by air to the oxide. Electropositive. Reacts with hydrogen on warming to form hydrides. Yields compounds on warming with group 5 and group 6 non-metals.	Kidney
Berkelium	The same as Curium	Bladder
Californium	The same as Curium	Large Intestine
Einsteinium	The same as Curium	Heart
Fermium	The same as Curium	Liver
Mendelevum	The same as Curium	Heart
Nobalium	The same as Curium	All
Lawrencium	The same as Curium	Kidney

The Lanthanides work against the destroying power of the Luziferic demons and their magnetic effect. The symptoms usually manifest in the soul body, in the astral body, in the chemical ether power. There are also 15 lanthanides, just as there are about 15 main groups of Luziferic entities/demons;

Lanthanium	Colourless	Spleen
	The Lanthanides were first discovered in 1787 when a unusual black mineral was found in Ytterby, Sweden. This mineral, now known as Gadolinite, was later separated into the various Lanthanide elements. In 1794, Professor Gadolin obtained yttria, an impure form of yttrium oxide, from the mineral. In 1803, Berzelius and Klaproth secluded the first Cerium compound. Later, Moseley used an x-ray-spectra of the elements to prove that there were fourteen elements between Lanthanum and Hafnium. The rest of the elements were later separated from the same mineral. These elements were first classified as 'rare earth' due to the fact that obtained by reasonably rare minerals. However, this is can be misleading since the Lanthanide elements have a practically unlimited abundance. The term Lanthanides was adopted, originating from the first element of the series, Lanthanum.	
Cerium	Colourless	Spleen
	Discovered by Berzelius and Hisinger in 1803, but not isolated as a metal until 1875, cerium (named for the asteroid Ceres) is the most abundant of the so-called rare-earth metals. It begins the series of lanthanides that runs from elements 58 to 71. In pure form the element is a malleable and ductile metal, similar in coloring to	

	iron. It is much more reactive than iron, however, readily oxidizing in moist air and releasing hydrogen from boiling water. Friction from abrading a sample can cause it to ignite. Although the metal itself is too reactive for most uses, compounds of cerium are used in glass making and photography. It has limited use in some special alloys as well. Most commercial grade cerium is derived from monazite sand, which is a mixture of phosphates of many of the rare earth metals along with calcium and thorium.	
Praseodym	**Green** Praseodymium, which is named from the Greek prasios + didymos (green twin), was isolated and identified by von Welsbach in 1885 from what was known at the time as didymium. von Welsbach's work revealed that this "substance" actually contained two new elements, one of which was praseodymium (neodymium was the other). Pure praseodymium is silvery-white and fairly soft. It oxidizes slowly in air and reacts vigorously with water to release hydrogen gas. It is used as an alloying agent along with magnesium for parts in aircraft engines. Misch metal is 5% praseodymium and is used for alloying steel and in flints used to create sparks in lighters. The glass in welder's goggles contains a mixture of praseodymium and neodymium.	**Lung**
Neodymium	**Red** Discovered in 1885 along with praseodymium, neodymium is named from the Greek neos + didymos (new twin). The silvery-white metal oxidizes easily in air and reacts with water, displacing hydrogen gas. Although another of the "rare" earth metals,	**Lung & kidney**

	neodymium is actually more abundant than many better known metals such as gold, silver, tin and lead. Misch metal, used in lighter flints, is about 18% neodymium. The element is also used in the manufacture of artificial rubies for laser applications.	
Prometium	**yellow** The existence of promethium (for the Greek god, Promethius) was predicted in 1912 when Henry Moseley developed an x-ray method for determining integer atomic numbers of elements. An element was clearly missing between neodymium and samarium. It's existence was not confirmed until 1947 by Marinsky, Glendenin and Coryell. Historical claims for the discovery of element 61 create an interesting trail from around 1925 in Florence (suggested name: florentium) to America in 1926 (suggested name: illinium). None of the claims, however, could be substantiated and today we know they were not simply a result of fleetingly small samples but rather poor work. While spectral lines of promethium are evident in the light from some stars, it now seems apparent that no promethium is found in accessible areas of the earth--hence the difficulty in finding any! Initial attempts at synthesis of element 61 in a cyclotron at Ohio State University in 1941 led to the suggested name cyclonium. But the recognized synthesis and identification finally came at Oak Ridge in 1947. The longest-lived isotope of promethium is Pm-145 with a half-life of 17.7 years. There are no significant commercial uses of the metal and so very little has been produced except for theoretical studies.	KIDNEY

Samarium	Yellow	Liver
	Named for the mineral samarskite from which it is extracted, samarium was isolated and identified by de Boisbaudran is 1879. The pure metal has a silver lustre and tarnishes slowly at room conditions. It is readily magnetized and holds its magnetism extremely well. Rare earth magnets (samarium-cobalt, for example) exploit this property. Although it is present in samarskite, commercial production of samarium is from monazite sand which can contain as much as 2.8% Sm by weight.	
Europium	Pink	Heart
	Europium looks and feels a lot like lead, although it is not as dense. It was discovered in 1896, and isolated in 1901 by Demarcay, working with samples of supposedly "pure" samarium. Named for the continent of Europe, the element ranks thirteenth in abundance among the rare earth metals, but there is more of it than silver and gold combined. It is the most reactive of the rare earth metals, behaving with water in a manner similar to calcium. Generally refined from monazite sand, the pure metal has few applications, but you would find it less interesting to read this without some of its compounds, which are used as activators and red phosphors in color CRT screens for television and computers.	
Gadolinium	Colourless	Kidney
	Gadolinium (from the mineral gadolinite, named for the Finnish chemist Gadolin) is a soft silvery-white metal that is used as an alloying agent in some steels and in the manufacture	

	of some electronic components. Credit for its discovery is shared by de Marignac who did extensive spectroscopic studies on the mixture then known as didymia, and by de Boisbaudran who finally isolated the metal in 1886. The metal has a very large capacity for absorbing thermal neutrons, making it an excellent material for control rods in fission power plants.	
Terbium	Pink Terbium is fourteenth in abundance among the 17 metals usually counted as "rare-earths", present in the earth's crust to the extent of only 0.9 ppm (about 1 teaspoon in every 63 tons of earth). Named for the Swedish village of Ytterby, the metal was discovered in 1843 by Mosander (along with erbium). Small amounts of terbium are used in special lasers and some solid state devices. The monazite sand from which terbium is generally extracted contains only about 0.03% by weight of Tb.	Lung
Dysprosium	Yellow The Greek word dysprositos (hard to get at) gives some indication of the scarcity of dysprosium, but only to a degree. It is about twice as abundant as uranium. The soft, silvery metal was discovered by de Boisbaudran in 1886 and it was finally isolated in 1906 by Urbain. A pure sample was not produced until the 1950s. The pure metal oxidizes readily in air.	Hidden lung
Holmium	Yellow Holmium was discovered by Cleve in 1879 and named for the Latinized version of the name for Stockholm. Like most of the other rare-earth	Heart

	metals, it is silvery and soft, and can be pounded or rolled into very thin sheets. At normal temperatures it is fairly inert but will oxidize at high temperatures and humidities. Like most of the rare-earth metals, holmium is generally obtained from monazite sand, where it is present to the extent of about 0.05%. Most holmium use is confined to research.	
Erbium	Red	Kidney
	Like the histories of the discoveries of many other rare-earths, the tale of erbium reads like a series of mistaken identities. These elements are generally found as oxides and most often together. Chemically, the oxides are very similar and at the time of their first examination were difficult to separate. Thus a sample of "lanthanum" might end up containing two additional elements that no one had bothered to look for. Many chemists thought that the oxides were elements themselves at one time. The oxide of yttrium (which along with scandium and lanthanum is generally included with the "rare-earths") known as yttria was eventually found to contain erbia and terbia as well, the oxides of, respectively, erbium and terbium. But the two are so similar that they were often confused in early work and what we now call erbium was originally terbium! In both cases, the credit for discovery goes to Mosander (1843 for erbium) and both elements were named for the Swedish town of Ytterby (which, by the way, also lends its name to Ytterbium and Yttrium----certainly some kind of record where naming elements is concerned!). Like most of the rare-earth metals, erbium is silvery and soft, tarnishing slightly in air.	

Thulium	Green	Spleen
	The rarest of the naturally-occurring rare-earth metals, thulium was discovered in 1879 by Cleve, working from samples of erbia, an oxide of erbium. The metal is named for the ancient name for Scandinavia, Thule. Like others in the lanthanide series, thulium is silver in color but it is also very soft---soft enough to cut with a knife.	
Ytterbium	Colourless	Spleen
	The first of the so-called "rare-earths" to be discovered, ytterbium takes its name from the Swedish village Ytterby (also the source of the names for terbium, erbium and yttrium). Discovery is credited to de Marignac in 1878. Initial identification was tediously made from the same mixture that most chemists of the time worked from: oxides of the lanthanides which gave rise to the term "rare-earth" due to its powdery consistency and often brownish color. But with the chemical separation techniques available at the time, it was very difficult to distinguish these similar elements. Even ytterbium itself turned out to hide another element. Lutetium was separated from it in 1907. Pure ytterbium is like most of the lanthanides: silvery and ductile, reacting slowly with air to form an oxide. Mostly obtained from monazite sand, ytterbium makes up about 0.03% of that mixture.	
Lutetium	Colourless	Spleen
	Lutetium ranks among the rare-earths in abundance only above thulium and promethium (and there's none of that anyway!). It official name comes from an ancient name for Paris, Lutecia, but	

it has had many names, most recently lutecium (only a change in official spelling). It was discovered independently by von Welsbach and Urbain in 1907-08.The refinement of ion exchange methods and their application to the separation of the rare-earths made the separation of lutetium from ytterbium possible. von Welsbach decided to rename ytterbium aldebaranium and picked cassiopium for element 71. Urbain preferred neoytterbium and lutecium. Urbain's choices eventually were accepted, altho

ugh the prefix was dropped from ytterbium and the spelling of lutecium was eventually changed.The metal is the hardest and densest of the rare-earths and is the last of the lanthanides.

The Metals work against the destroying power of the Ahrimanic demons, through their relation to electricity. They demolish the light ether. The symptoms are often in the etheric body. There are 7 main metals, as there are 7 main planets that support the 7 main organs;

1. Mercurius, protects the intestines from the influence of Ahrimanic powers.
2. Cuprum, protects the reproductive organs from the influence of Ahrimanic powers.
3. Argentum, protects the kidneys from the influence of Ahrimanic powers.
4. Aurum, protects the heart from the influence of Ahrimanic powers.
5. Ferrum, protects the gall-bladder from the influence of Ahrimanic powers.
6. Stannum, protects the liver from the influence of Ahrimanic powers.
7. Plumbum, protects the spleen from the influence of Ahrimanic powers.

An observation concerning the Actinides and the Lanthanides;

There are 15 Lanthanides and 15 Actinides. They mirror each other in a special and peculiar way.

- Firstly the second half of the 15 Actinides mirror in reverse order the first part (1=15, 2=14 and so on).
- Secondly the second half of the 15 Lanthanides mirror in reverse order the first part (1=15, 2=14 and so on).
- Thirdly the whole row of Actinides mirror the whole row of Lanthanides and vica versa.

Numbers 1 and 2 relate to earth, to the spleen. Then lung and kidney are related to number 5. The balancing middle numbers 7-8 are lung in the Actinides and heart in the Lanthanides.

So then we start on the «descending» part. The next one after the balancing middle point is then kidney, number 8 in each row, mirroring number 5-6. Then number 10 expresses lung, mirroring number 4. Number 11 expresses itself in both rows as heart, mirroring number 3, but here expressed in a Controlling cycle as lung. Why this is so I do not know.

Then something interesting appears. In the Lanthanides the last three; 13, 14, 15, express the earth, the spleen, while in the Actinides they express all the organ-processes.

The Lanthanides expresses the fight against the demons that attack the astral body, the Luziferic demons.

The Actinides express or activate the fight against the demons that attack the «I», the Azuras.

The Lanthanides were found in 1787, when the fight against the Luziferic demons excelerated[5].

---

[5] See more of this in the writings of Rudolf Steiner

The Actinides were mostly found in the 20. century[6], as the fight for the human I excelerated.

---

[6] *Uranium and thorium were the first actinides discovered. Uranium was identified in 1789 by the German chemist Martin Heinrich Klaproth in pitchblende ore. He named it after the planet Uranus which had been discovered only eight years earlier. Klaproth was able to precipitate a yellow compound (likely sodium diuranate) by dissolving pitchblende in nitric acid and neutralizing the solution with sodium hydroxide. He then reduced the obtained yellow powder with charcoal, and extracted a black substance that he mistook for metal. Only 60 years later, the French scientist Eugène-Melchior Péligot identified it with uranium oxide. He also isolated the first sample of uranium metal by heating uranium tetrachloride with potassium. The atomic mass of uranium was then calculated as 120, but Dmitri Mendeleev in 1872 corrected it to 240 using his periodicity laws. This value was confirmed experimentally in 1882 by K. Zimmerman. Thorium oxide was discovered by Friedrich Wöhler in the mineral, which was found in Norway (1827). Jöns Jacob Berzelius characterized this material in more detail by in 1828. By reduction of thorium tetrachloride with potassium, he isolated the metal and named it thorium after the Norse god of thunder and lightning Thor. The same isolation method was later used by Péligot for uranium. Actinium was discovered in 1899 by André-Louis Debierne, an assistant of Marie Curie, in the pitchblende waste left after removal of radium and polonium. He described the substance (in 1899) as similar to titanium and (in 1900) as similar to thorium. The discovery of actinium by Debierne was however questioned in 1971 and 2000, arguing that Debierne's publications in 1904 contradicted his earlier work of 1899–1900. The name actinium comes from the Greek aktis, aktinos (ακτίς, ακτίνος), meaning beam or ray. This metal was discovered not by its own radiation but by the radiation of the daughter products. Owing to the close similarity of actinium and lanthanum and low abundance, pure actinium could only be produced in 1950. The term actinide was probably introduced by Victor Goldschmidt in 1937. Protactinium was possibly isolated in 1900 by William Crookes. It was first identified in 1913, when Kasimir Fajans and Oswald Helmuth Göhring encountered the short-lived isotope ^{234m}Pa (half-life 1.17 minutes) during their studies of the ^{238}U decay. They named the new element brevium (from Latin brevis meaning brief); the name was changed to protoactinium (from Greek πρῶτος + ἀκτίς meaning "first beam element") in 1918 when two groups of scientists, led by the Austrian Lise Meitner and Otto Hahn of Germany and Frederick Soddy and John Cranston of Great Britain, independently discovered ^{231}Pa. The name was shortened to protactinium in 1949. This element was little characterized until 1960, when A. G. Maddock and his co-workers in the U.K. produced 130 grams of protactinium from 60 tonnes of waste left after extraction of uranium from its ore.*

Grundstoffernes Periodiske Syste

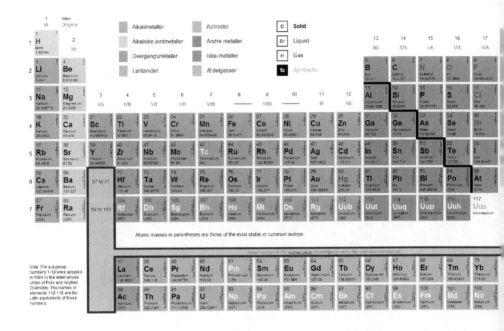

Atomic masses in parentheses are those of the most stable or common isotope

Note. The subgroup
numbers 1-18 were adopted
in 1984 by the International
Union of Pure and Applied
Chemistry. The names of
elements 112-118 are the
Latin equivalents of those
numbers.

Closing remarks;

A Resurrection.

In my first book[7] I wrote a closing remark entiteled "Requiem". The conclusion was as follows; .....

"We have come together in a journey of knowledge to the last page, the end of the "active life" of this book. By now, you should have spent several hours reading this work. If you have not done so, please go back and read it again before you proceed! One spoils the enjoyment of a thriller if one reads the last page first! I want you to read this requiem only when you have grasped the ideas in this book and you have made its thinking process an instinctive part of your thinking process.

A requiem is a formal farewell ceremony for the dead. In its briefest form, it can be a note on a grave, or tomb. It points beyond the grave, beyond death, to the afterlife. In the Christian tradition, the most common requiem is "Requiescant in Pacem" – "May they rest in Peace".

In a certain sense, with these last words I want to demolish all that I have said in this book, but also show the necessity of its writing. As life that dies in the leaf fall of autumn resurrects in the green shoots of spring, this requiem shows how all that has been written in this book will resurrect in a new way, in a new life of meaning and context.

The intricate medical or healing systems that we have made and believe in, do not work in or of themselves. The most important component of healing is our own will and intention, which can kindle belief of the patient and auto-cure, i.e. the healing capacity of the body itself. Most people reject the idea that an animal's "belief" (if there is such a faculty) could have anything to do with clinical

---

[7] *Holistic Veterinary Medicine, Amazon, ISBN 10-1467991104*

results. However, animal owners, and most good veterinarians (whether conventional or holistic) know that animals have highly developed instincts to distinguish "friend" from "foe". It is uncanny how often animals sense the good intentions of a holistic veterinarian. They usually respond by allowing handling or other interventions, such as multiple needling or spinal manipulations that would put many conventional veterinarians in great danger of being bitten, scratched or kicked! Holistic veterinarians know that animals see them as "friend". This intention, will and courage to cure and heal, also carries the potential to heal, or start the patients self healing abilities to cure themselves. As two of my teachers have said:

- "If you can really visualize the effects of a point, you need not insert a needle" (Georg Bentze)
- "If you really know the workings of a homeopathic remedy, it is enough to think that you give it to a patient" (Margit Engel).

The concepts in this book are absent from, or hard to find in other books. However, these concepts are very important for professionals who want to improve their clinical success rates. When you have assimilated it and made it real for yourself, it becomes superfluous to your needs and you can dismiss it. When this happens, it resurrects as your own healing, intuitive powers. Then you become a true healer.

I most earnestly invite you to try these methods with an open mind and an honest, loving heart".

#

In this book I have deepened and elaborated on this, bringing the conclusion a step further.

A conclusion of the Requiem.

And the conclusion of the Requiem is the Resurrection.
As Christianity is nothing without the resurrection, healing is nothing without the solution of the translocation. It must be realized that life is spiritual, as are diseases.

When this fundamental fact becomes part of our understanding, we become true healers.

Acknowledgement;

Thanking my colleges and inspirators

Man does not live alone in the world.

This book would have been impossible to write without the inspirations and advices from close friends and colleges as;

Tierheilpraktiker Corinne Dettmer, Dr. Med. Vet. Markus Steiner, nurse Margit Buen, artist Philip Nordtvedt,
Dr. Vet. Prof. Bruce Ferguson, Dr. Ferdinand Niessen,
Agronomist Asbjørn Lavoll and artist Lizz Daniels.

Thank you to all.

31098535R00053

Made in the USA
Middletown, DE
28 December 2018